HEARTBEATS AND HEALTH

THE SOCIETAL IMPLICATIONS OF HYPERTENSION

BY
MICHEL
MONTALVO

Table of Contents

- Introduction
- Understanding Hypertension
- Causes and Contributors
- Health Consequences of Hypertension
- Economic and Social Impact
- Cultural Perspectives on Hypertension
- Awareness and Education
- Prevention and Management Strategies
- Technological Innovations
- Future Directions and Research
- Conclusion
- Resources and Further Reading
- References

Chapter I
Introduction
Overview of Hypertension

Hypertension, commonly known as high blood pressure, is a condition where the force of blood against the artery walls is consistently too high. It is often called a "silent killer" because it typically has no symptoms until significant damage has been done. Blood pressure is measured in millimeters of mercury (mmHg) and is expressed as two numbers: systolic (the pressure when the heart beats) over diastolic (the pressure when the heart rests between beats). A normal blood pressure reading is typically around 120/80 mmHg; hypertension is diagnosed when readings consistently exceed 130/80 mmHg.

Prevalence and Importance

According to the World Health Organization (WHO), hypertension affects over 1.5 billion people globally and is a leading risk factor for heart disease, stroke, and premature death. Its rising prevalence, driven by lifestyle changes, urbanization, and aging populations, poses significant public health challenges. Understanding hypertension is crucial for developing effective strategies for prevention, management, and education.

Purpose of the book

This ebook aims to explore the multifaceted implications of hypertension on individuals and society as a whole. It seeks to provide readers with a comprehensive understanding of the condition, from its causes and health consequences to its economic and social impacts. By highlighting the stories of those affected, we aim to humanize the statistics and foster a greater sense of urgency in addressing this health crisis.

Chapter II
Understanding Hypertension Defining the Condition and Its Classifications

Hypertension, or high blood pressure, is a chronic medical condition characterized by elevated pressure within the arteries. Blood pressure is the force exerted by circulating blood against the walls of the body's arteries, which is essential for maintaining blood flow to organs and tissues. Blood pressure readings consist of two measurements:

- Systolic Blood Pressure (SBP): The higher number, which measures the pressure in the arteries when the heart beats and pumps blood.
- Diastolic Blood Pressure (DBP): The lower number, which measures the pressure in the arteries when the heart is at rest between beats.

A typical normal blood pressure reading is around 120/80 mmHg. Hypertension is generally diagnosed when blood pressure readings consistently exceed 130/80 mmHg, according to guidelines set by organizations such as the American College of Cardiology and the American Heart Association.

NORMAL	LESS THAN 120	and	LESS THAN 80
ELEVATED	120 – 129	and	LESS THAN 80
HIGH BLOOD PRESSURE (HYPERTENSION) STAGE 1	130 – 139	or	80 – 89
HIGH BLOOD PRESSURE (HYPERTENSION) STAGE 2	140 OR HIGHER	or	90 OR HIGHER
HYPERTENSIVE CRISIS (consult your doctor immediately)	HIGHER THAN 180	and/or	HIGHER THAN 120

Classifications of Hypertension

Hypertension is classified into several categories based on the severity of the condition:

1. **Primary (Essential) Hypertension:**
   - This is the most common form of hypertension, accounting for approximately 90-95% of all cases.
   - Primary hypertension develops gradually over many years and is typically attributed to a combination of genetic, environmental, and lifestyle factors.
   - Common risk factors include obesity, a sedentary lifestyle, high salt intake, and stress.

2. **Secondary Hypertension:**

- This form is less common and occurs as a result of an underlying health condition.
- Secondary hypertension can develop suddenly and cause higher blood pressure than primary hypertension.
- Causes may include kidney disease, hormonal disorders (such as hyperthyroidism or Cushing's syndrome), certain medications, and sleep apnea.

3. **Isolated Systolic Hypertension:**

- This occurs when the systolic blood pressure is elevated (typically above 130 mmHg) while the diastolic pressure remains normal (less than 80 mmHg).
- Isolated systolic hypertension is more common in older adults and is often associated with stiffness in the arteries.

4. Malignant Hypertension:

- A severe form of hypertension that can lead to organ damage and is characterized by extremely high blood pressure readings, usually above 180/120 mmHg.
- This condition requires immediate medical intervention to prevent life-threatening complications.

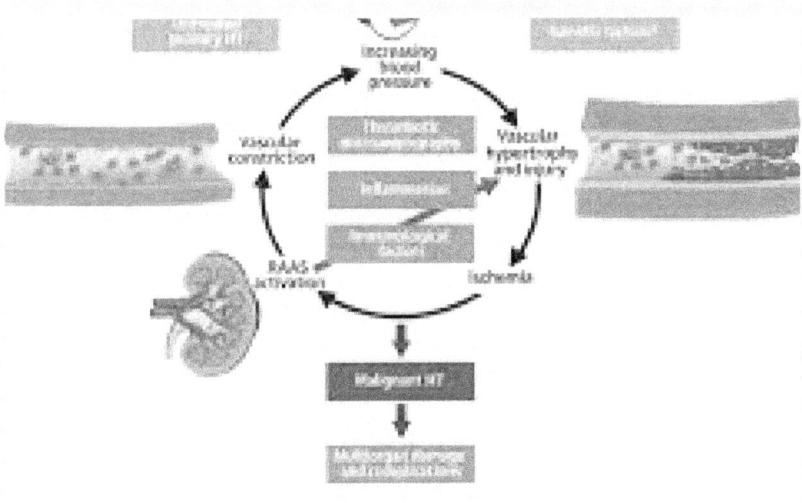

okestreka R, et al. J Am Coll Cardiol. 2024;83(17):1688-1701.

5. **Hypertensive Crisis:**

- This is an acute and severe increase in blood pressure that can be classified into two types:
    - Hypertensive Urgency: Blood pressure is extremely high (generally above 180/120 mmHg) but without acute organ damage. This condition requires prompt medical evaluation and management.
    - Hypertensive Emergency: Blood pressure is similarly high, but there are signs of organ damage, such as chest pain, shortness of breath, or neurological symptoms. This situation requires immediate medical attention.

Conclusion

Understanding hypertension and its classifications is crucial for effective diagnosis and management. Each type of hypertension may require different approaches to treatment and lifestyle modifications. Recognizing the nuances of this condition can empower individuals to take proactive steps toward their health, engage with healthcare providers, and advocate for better management strategies. As we continue to explore the causes and implications of hypertension, it becomes evident that awareness and education are key components in combating this prevalent health issue.

Chapter III
Causes and Contributors

Hypertension is a complex condition influenced by a variety of factors, both modifiable and non-modifiable. Understanding these causes is essential for effective prevention and management. This section explores the key contributors to hypertension, categorizing them into lifestyle factors, genetic predispositions, and environmental influences.

1. **Lifestyle Factors**

Diet and Nutrition:
- High Sodium Intake: Excessive salt consumption is one of the leading dietary contributors to hypertension. Sodium can cause the body to retain water, increasing blood volume and, consequently, blood pressure. The World Health Organization recommends limiting sodium intake to less than 2,000 mg per day.
- Low Potassium Intake: Potassium helps balance sodium levels in the body. A diet rich in fruits and vegetables can help lower blood pressure, while inadequate potassium can exacerbate hypertension.
- Processed Foods: Many processed and fast foods are high in sodium and unhealthy fats, contributing to weight gain and increased blood pressure.

b. **Physical Inactivity:**

- Sedentary lifestyles are a significant risk factor for hypertension. Regular physical activity strengthens the heart, enabling it to pump blood more efficiently and reducing the pressure in the arteries.
- Aim for at least 150 minutes of moderate aerobic exercise or 75 minutes of vigorous exercise each week to maintain a healthy blood pressure.

c. **Stress:**

- Chronic stress may contribute to hypertension through mechanisms such as hormonal changes and unhealthy coping behaviors (e.g., overeating, smoking, or increased alcohol consumption).

- Stress management techniques, including mindfulness, meditation, and regular exercise, can help mitigate its impact on blood pressure.

d. **Tobacco and Alcohol Use:**

- Tobacco: Smoking damages blood vessels and raises blood pressure. Even secondhand smoke can contribute to hypertension.

- Alcohol: While moderate alcohol consumption may have some cardiovascular benefits, excessive drinking can raise blood pressure significantly. The American Heart Association recommends limiting alcohol to one drink per day for women and two drinks for men.

2. Genetic Predispositions

Genetics plays a significant role in the development of hypertension. Individuals with a family history of high blood pressure are at a higher risk of developing the condition themselves. Certain genetic variations can affect how the body regulates blood pressure, including how it processes sodium, manages stress hormones, and maintains blood vessel health.

Research continues to uncover specific genes associated with hypertension, leading to a better understanding of the biological mechanisms involved. This knowledge can inform personalized approaches to prevention and treatment.

3. **Environmental Influences**

a. Urbanization:

- Rapid urbanization often leads to lifestyle changes, including increased consumption of processed foods, decreased physical activity, and heightened stress levels, all of which contribute to hypertension.

- Urban environments can also expose individuals to higher levels of air pollution, which has been linked to increased blood pressure.

b. **Socioeconomic Factors:**

- Lower socioeconomic status is associated with higher rates of hypertension. Limited access to healthy foods, healthcare services, and opportunities for physical activity can exacerbate health disparities.

- Education and awareness play critical roles in managing hypertension, as individuals in higher socioeconomic brackets often have better access to information and resources.

c. **Sleep Quality:**

- Poor sleep quality and conditions like sleep apnea can significantly affect blood pressure. Interrupted sleep patterns can lead to increased stress hormones, weight gain, and ultimately, higher blood pressure.

- Prioritizing sleep hygiene and seeking treatment for sleep disorders are essential for maintaining healthy blood pressure levels.

Conclusion

Hypertension is influenced by a myriad of factors that interconnect in complex ways. Understanding the causes and contributors to this condition empowers individuals to make informed lifestyle choices and seek appropriate medical guidance. By addressing modifiable risk factors—such as diet, exercise, and stress management—along with recognizing genetic and environmental influences, we can work towards reducing the prevalence of hypertension and improving overall public health.

Chapter IV
Health Consequences of Hypertension

Hypertension is often referred to as a **"silent killer"** because it can progress for years without noticeable symptoms, yet it significantly increases the risk of serious health complications. Understanding the health consequences of hypertension is crucial for recognizing its impact not only on individual well-being but also on overall public health. This section will explore the short-term and long-term effects of high blood pressure, the comorbidities associated with the condition, and its impact on quality of life.

1. **Short-term Effects**

While many people may not experience immediate symptoms, some individuals may encounter short-term effects that can be alarming. These may include:

- Headaches: Some people report experiencing headaches, especially during hypertensive crises, when blood pressure spikes to dangerously high levels.

- Dizziness or Lightheadedness: Fluctuations in blood pressure can lead to episodes of dizziness, especially when standing up quickly.

- Nosebleeds: Though relatively rare, sudden increases in blood pressure can lead to nosebleeds in some individuals.

- Visual Disturbances: High blood pressure can cause blurred vision or other visual disturbances, particularly in severe cases.

These symptoms can serve as warning signs that prompt individuals to seek medical attention, highlighting the importance of regular monitoring and awareness.

2. **Long-term Effects**

If left unmanaged, hypertension can lead to a range of serious health complications over time:
- Heart Disease: High blood pressure is a major risk factor for coronary artery disease, heart attacks, and heart failure. The increased pressure can cause the heart to work harder, leading to left ventricular hypertrophy (enlargement of the heart) and eventually heart failure.
- Stroke: Hypertension significantly raises the risk of both ischemic (caused by blocked blood vessels) and hemorrhagic (caused by bleeding in the brain) strokes. It can weaken blood vessels in the brain, making them more susceptible to rupture or blockage.

- Kidney Damage: The kidneys play a crucial role in regulating blood pressure. Chronic hypertension can damage the blood vessels in the kidneys, leading to chronic kidney disease (CKD) or even kidney failure. Managing blood pressure is essential to preserving kidney function.

- Vision Loss: High blood pressure can cause damage to the blood vessels in the eyes, leading to hypertensive retinopathy, which can result in vision impairment or loss. Regular eye exams are important for monitoring eye health in individuals with hypertension.

- Aneurysms: Prolonged high blood pressure can weaken blood vessels and increase the risk of aneurysms—abnormal bulges in the walls of blood vessels. If an aneurysm ruptures, it can lead to life-threatening internal bleeding.

- Metabolic Syndrome: Hypertension is a key component of metabolic syndrome, a cluster of conditions that includes obesity, high blood sugar, and abnormal cholesterol levels. This syndrome increases the risk of heart disease, stroke, and diabetes.

3. Comorbidities Associated with Hypertension

Hypertension often coexists with other medical conditions, exacerbating health risks:

- Diabetes: There is a strong correlation between hypertension and diabetes. Individuals with diabetes are more likely to develop high blood pressure due to insulin resistance and metabolic changes. Conversely, hypertension increases the risk of diabetes-related complications.

- Obesity: Excess weight increases the likelihood of developing hypertension. Fat tissue can produce hormones that increase blood pressure, while the additional strain on the cardiovascular system exacerbates the condition.

- Sleep Apnea: This sleep disorder, characterized by interrupted breathing during sleep, is common among individuals with hypertension. It can contribute to elevated blood pressure levels and create a vicious cycle of worsening health.

4. Impact on Quality of Life

Beyond the physical health consequences, hypertension can also affect an individual's overall quality of life:

- **Mental Health:** Living with hypertension can lead to increased anxiety and stress, particularly concerning the potential for serious health complications. Individuals may experience feelings of helplessness or fear related to their condition.

- Lifestyle Limitations: The need for ongoing medical management and lifestyle changes (such as dietary restrictions and exercise) can be challenging and may lead to frustration or social withdrawal.

- Financial Burden: The costs associated with managing hypertension, including medications, regular check-ups, and potential hospitalizations, can create a significant financial burden for individuals and families.

Conclusion

Hypertension is not merely a number on a medical chart; it is a condition with profound implications for individual health and well-being. Understanding the short-term and long-term health consequences of hypertension underscores the importance of proactive management and lifestyle modifications. By recognizing the risks associated with high blood pressure, individuals can take meaningful steps toward improving their health outcomes and enhancing their quality of life.

Chapter V

Economic and Social Impact of Hypertension

Hypertension is not only a significant health concern but also a pressing economic and social issue that affects individuals, families, and communities at large. Understanding its broader implications is essential for addressing the challenges it presents. This section explores the financial burden of hypertension on healthcare systems, its impact on workforce productivity, and the broader societal effects.

1. **Healthcare Costs Associated with Hypertension**

The economic burden of hypertension is substantial, encompassing both direct and indirect costs:

a. Direct Medical Expenses:
- Treatment Costs: Managing hypertension often requires ongoing medical care, including regular doctor visits, diagnostic tests, and medication. The costs associated with antihypertensive drugs can add up significantly over time, especially for individuals requiring multiple medications.

Emergency Care and Hospitalization:

- Uncontrolled hypertension can lead to serious complications such as heart attacks and strokes, resulting in emergency room visits and hospital stays, which further inflate healthcare costs. According to various studies, hospitalization due to hypertension-related complications can exceed thousands of dollars per incident.

b. **Indirect Costs:**

- Lost Productivity: Individuals with hypertension may experience absenteeism (missing work) or presenteeism (being present but not fully functional at work) due to health issues. This loss of productivity can have cascading effects on businesses and the economy. It is estimated that the economic costs associated with lost productivity due to hypertension run into billions of dollars annually.
- Long-term Disability: Severe complications from hypertension, such as heart failure or stroke, can lead to long-term disability, reducing the ability to work and increasing dependency on social services and disability benefits.

2. **Impact on Workforce Productivity**

Hypertension poses significant challenges in the workplace, affecting both employees and employers:
a. Employee Well-Being:

- Health issues stemming from hypertension can diminish an employee's overall quality of life, leading to decreased job satisfaction and lower morale. Chronic health problems can create a cycle of stress that exacerbates both hypertension and workplace performance.

b. **Employer Costs:**

- Companies may incur higher insurance premiums and healthcare costs due to increased claims related to hypertension and its complications. Implementing wellness programs and preventative measures can be an effective strategy for reducing overall healthcare costs.

c. Worksite Interventions:
- Employers that prioritize employee health through interventions such as health screenings, fitness programs, and stress management resources can enhance workforce productivity and reduce the economic burden associated with hypertension.

3. Societal Effects and Health Disparities

The societal impact of hypertension extends beyond economic costs:

a. Health Disparities:

- Hypertension disproportionately affects low-income populations and marginalized communities. Factors such as limited access to healthcare, poor nutrition, and lack of education contribute to higher rates of hypertension in these groups. Addressing these disparities is critical for promoting health equity and improving overall community health.

b. **Public Health Implications:**
- The prevalence of hypertension can strain public health resources, leading to increased demand for healthcare services, which can overwhelm existing systems. This situation necessitates a coordinated response from public health authorities, healthcare providers, and policymakers.

c. Community Resources:
- Communities with high rates of hypertension may face broader social challenges, such as increased healthcare costs and reduced economic productivity. Efforts to promote community health through education, access to healthy foods, and physical activity programs are essential for combating hypertension at the community level.

4. **Future Considerations**

Addressing the economic and social impact of hypertension requires a multifaceted approach:

- Policy Interventions: Governments and health organizations must develop policies that promote access to preventive care, education, and resources for managing hypertension. This can include funding for community health initiatives and public awareness campaigns.

Education and Awareness:

- Increasing awareness of hypertension's risk factors, management strategies, and consequences is vital. Educational programs in schools and workplaces can empower individuals to make healthier lifestyle choices.

- Collaboration Across Sectors: A holistic approach that involves collaboration between healthcare providers, employers, community organizations, and policymakers can create supportive environments that facilitate better health outcomes.

Conclusion

Hypertension is a complex condition that carries significant economic and social implications. By understanding these impacts, we can better advocate for effective prevention and management strategies, reduce health disparities, and enhance overall community well-being. Addressing hypertension requires collective action and commitment from individuals, healthcare systems, and society as a whole.

Chapter VI
Cultural Perspectives on Hypertension

Hypertension is a global health issue, but its perception, understanding, and management can vary significantly across different cultures. Cultural beliefs, dietary habits, healthcare practices, and societal norms all influence how hypertension is viewed and treated. This section explores the diverse cultural perspectives on hypertension, highlighting how these factors shape individual and community responses to the condition.

1. **Dietary Practices Across Cultures**

a. Traditional Diets:

- Dietary patterns play a crucial role in the prevalence and management of hypertension. For example, the Mediterranean diet, rich in fruits, vegetables, whole grains, and healthy fats, has been associated with lower blood pressure levels. In contrast, diets high in processed foods and sodium are prevalent in many Western cultures, contributing to increased rates of hypertension.

In Asian cultures, traditional diets often emphasize rice, fish, and vegetables, which may contribute to lower hypertension rates compared to Western diets. However, rapid urbanization and the adoption of Western eating habits in many Asian countries are leading to rising hypertension levels.

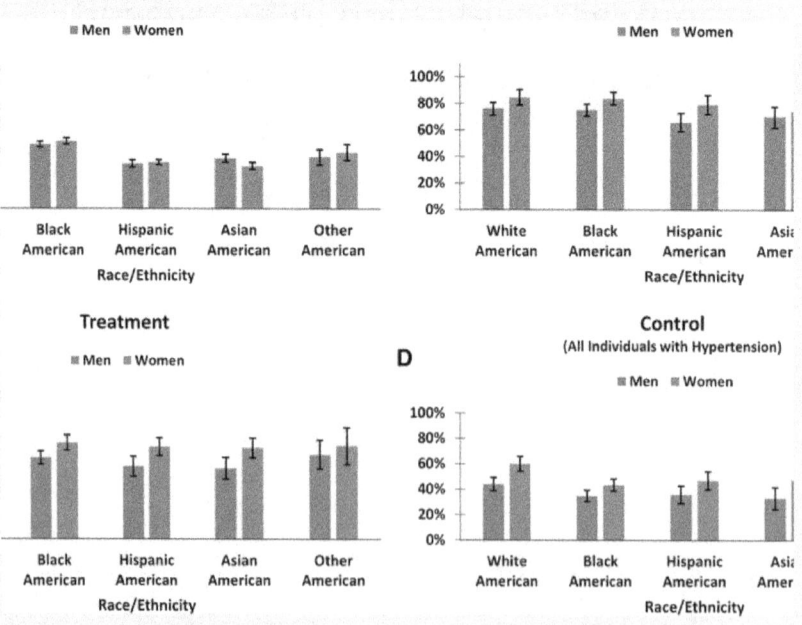

b. **Cultural Attitudes Toward Food:**

- Food serves as a significant cultural marker, with many societies placing a strong emphasis on communal meals and culinary traditions. In some cultures, high-sodium foods, such as fermented products or cured meats, are staples, which can pose risks for hypertension. Understanding these cultural dietary practices is essential for developing effective public health interventions that respect and incorporate local food traditions.

2. **Attitudes Towards Health and Illness**

a. Perception of Hypertension:
- In some cultures, hypertension may not be viewed as a serious health concern, particularly if symptoms are not immediately apparent. This can lead to delays in seeking treatment and management, as individuals may prioritize visible health issues over chronic conditions like hypertension.

- Conversely, in cultures where there is a strong emphasis on preventive healthcare, individuals may be more proactive about monitoring blood pressure and managing risk factors, reflecting a broader understanding of the importance of maintaining health.

b. **Stigma and Beliefs:**

- The cultural stigma surrounding chronic illnesses can affect how individuals approach hypertension. In some communities, there may be a belief that high blood pressure is a sign of weakness or failure, leading to reluctance in seeking help. Addressing these stigmas through education and awareness is crucial for improving health outcomes.

3. **Traditional and Alternative Treatments**

a. Herbal Remedies and Traditional Medicine:

- Many cultures have their traditional remedies for managing hypertension. In some African and Asian cultures, herbal treatments are commonly used, with plants like garlic, hibiscus, and ginger being popular choices. While some of these remedies may have beneficial effects on blood pressure, it is essential to ensure that individuals consult healthcare professionals before discontinuing prescribed medications.

Traditional healing practices often involve a holistic approach, considering the individual's physical, mental, and spiritual well-being. Integrating these practices with conventional medical treatments can enhance overall management strategies.

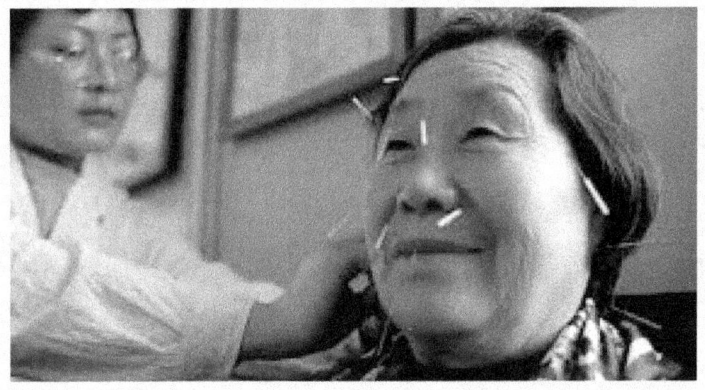

b. **Role of Community Health Workers:**

- In many cultures, community health workers play a vital role in educating individuals about hypertension and promoting healthy practices. These workers often have a deep understanding of local customs and beliefs, making them effective advocates for health promotion in their communities.

4. **Barriers to Accessing Healthcare**

a. Economic and Structural Barriers:
- Economic disparities can affect access to healthcare services and resources for managing hypertension. In low-income communities, individuals may struggle to afford medications or regular check-ups, exacerbating health inequalities.
- Cultural differences in healthcare utilization can also pose barriers. For instance, individuals from cultures that prioritize family and community care may be less likely to seek professional medical help, relying instead on traditional remedies or community support.

b. **Education and Awareness:**

- Limited health literacy can hinder individuals' understanding of hypertension and its management. Culturally tailored education programs that consider language, cultural beliefs, and practices are essential for effectively communicating the risks and treatment options for hypertension.

5. Globalization and Changing Perspectives

The process of globalization has led to significant changes in dietary habits, healthcare practices, and cultural beliefs worldwide. As societies adopt Western lifestyles, there is a growing incidence of hypertension in previously low-prevalence areas. This shift necessitates a nuanced understanding of how cultural factors influence health behaviors and the importance of preserving beneficial traditional practices while integrating modern medical approaches.

Conclusion

Cultural perspectives on hypertension significantly shape how individuals and communities understand, manage, and respond to this chronic condition. By recognizing the influence of cultural beliefs, dietary practices, and traditional remedies, healthcare providers and public health advocates can develop more effective, culturally sensitive strategies for prevention and management. Fostering awareness and education within diverse communities is vital for promoting healthier lifestyles and improving health outcomes related to hypertension.

Chapter 7
Awareness and Education

Effective awareness and education are critical components in the fight against hypertension. With a significant portion of the population unaware of their condition, and many individuals failing to understand the importance of management, fostering knowledge about hypertension can lead to better health outcomes. This section explores the current state of awareness, the importance of education, and strategies to enhance understanding of hypertension within communities.

1. **Current State of Awareness**

Despite the prevalence of hypertension, many individuals remain uninformed about the condition:
- Lack of Knowledge: Studies indicate that a substantial number of people with hypertension are unaware of their diagnosis. Many do not regularly monitor their blood pressure, leading to undetected and untreated conditions that can have serious health consequences.
- Misunderstanding Risk Factors: Many individuals do not fully grasp the risk factors associated with hypertension, such as lifestyle choices, family history, and environmental influences. This lack of understanding can prevent proactive measures to reduce risks.

2. The Importance of Education

Education plays a pivotal role in promoting health literacy, empowering individuals to take control of their health:
- Understanding Hypertension: Comprehensive education about what hypertension is, how it develops, and its potential health consequences can motivate individuals to seek regular check-ups and engage in healthy behaviors.
- Lifestyle Modifications: Educating individuals about dietary changes, physical activity, stress management, and the importance of medication adherence can significantly impact blood pressure control. Practical guidance on implementing these changes is crucial for success.

3. **Strategies for Enhancing Awareness**

To effectively promote awareness and education about hypertension, various strategies can be implemented:

a. Community Outreach Programs:
- Local health departments and community organizations can establish outreach programs to provide information about hypertension and its risks. These programs can include free blood pressure screenings, health fairs, and workshops that educate participants about prevention and management

b. **School-Based Education:**

- Incorporating health education into school curricula can instill knowledge about hypertension from a young age. Teaching students about healthy eating, the importance of physical activity, and stress management techniques can foster lifelong healthy habits.

c. Digital Campaigns:
- Utilizing social media and digital platforms can effectively reach a broad audience. Awareness campaigns that highlight risk factors, prevention strategies, and the importance of regular monitoring can engage individuals and encourage them to take action.

d. **Collaboration with Healthcare Providers:**

- Healthcare professionals play a crucial role in educating patients about hypertension. Providers can offer resources, conduct educational sessions during appointments, and create a supportive environment for patients to ask questions about their condition.

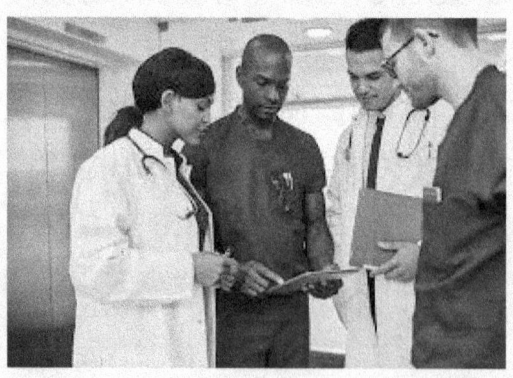

4. Cultural Competence in Education

To effectively reach diverse populations, education about hypertension must be culturally sensitive:

- Tailored Resources: Developing educational materials that are culturally relevant and available in multiple languages can enhance understanding and accessibility. This approach acknowledges the unique beliefs, practices, and challenges faced by different communities.
- Community Involvement: Engaging local leaders and community health workers in education efforts can build trust and encourage participation. These individuals can bridge cultural gaps and facilitate discussions about hypertension and health practices.

5. The Role of Technology

Advancements in technology provide new avenues for enhancing awareness and education:

- **Mobile Health Apps:** Health apps can empower individuals to monitor their blood pressure, track lifestyle changes, and receive reminders for medication adherence. Many apps also offer educational resources and articles about hypertension management.
- **Telehealth Services:** Telehealth allows individuals to connect with healthcare providers remotely, making it easier to access information and support. Virtual consultations can be particularly beneficial for those in underserved areas.

6. Measuring Impact

Evaluating the effectiveness of awareness and education initiatives is essential for continuous improvement:
- Surveys and Feedback: Conducting surveys before and after educational programs can provide insights into changes in knowledge and behaviors. Gathering feedback helps identify areas for improvement and tailor future initiatives.
- Community Health Metrics: Monitoring community health metrics, such as blood pressure levels and hospitalizations related to hypertension, can assess the overall impact of awareness efforts.

Conclusion

Awareness and education are fundamental to addressing the growing burden of hypertension. By empowering individuals with knowledge about the condition, its risk factors, and management strategies, we can foster healthier communities. Implementing culturally sensitive and accessible educational initiatives will create a stronger foundation for reducing the prevalence of hypertension and improving health outcomes for all.

Chapter VIII
Prevention and Management Strategies

Preventing and managing hypertension is essential for reducing its prevalence and minimizing associated health risks. Effective strategies encompass lifestyle modifications, medical interventions, and community support systems. This section outlines comprehensive approaches to both prevent and manage hypertension, empowering individuals to take control of their health.

1. **Lifestyle Modifications**

a. Dietary Changes:
   - DASH Diet: The Dietary Approaches to Stop Hypertension (DASH) diet emphasizes fruits, vegetables, whole grains, lean proteins, and low-fat dairy while reducing saturated fats and sodium intake. Studies have shown that following the DASH diet can significantly lower blood pressure.

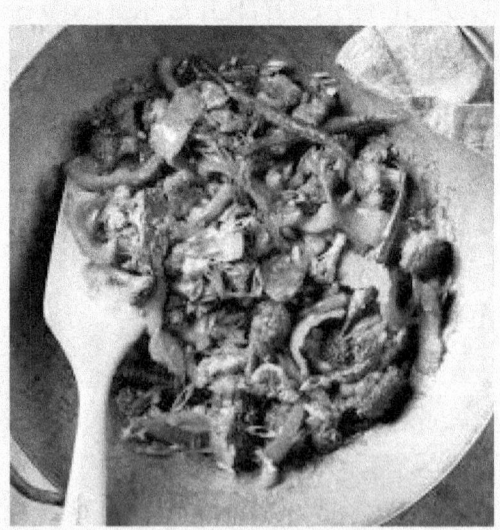

- **Sodium Reduction:**

- Reducing sodium intake is crucial. The American Heart Association recommends limiting sodium to no more than 2,300 mg per day, ideally aiming for 1,500 mg for optimal heart health. Reading food labels, avoiding processed foods, and using herbs and spices for flavor can aid in this effort.

- Increasing Potassium: Foods rich in potassium, such as bananas, oranges, spinach, and potatoes, can help balance sodium levels and lower blood pressure.

b. **Physical Activity:**

- Regular Exercise: Engaging in regular physical activity strengthens the heart and improves circulation. Aim for at least 150 minutes of moderate aerobic exercise or 75 minutes of vigorous exercise each week. Activities can include walking, cycling, swimming, or group fitness classes.
- Incorporating Movement: Simple changes, such as taking the stairs instead of the elevator, walking or biking for short trips, and incorporating stretching and strength training, can significantly contribute to overall physical activity levels.

c. **Weight Management:**

- Maintaining a Healthy Weight: Achieving and maintaining a healthy weight is vital for hypertension management. Even a modest weight loss of 5-10% can significantly lower blood pressure in overweight individuals.
- Balanced Nutrition: Combining dietary changes with regular physical activity is the most effective approach to weight management. Consulting with a registered dietitian can provide personalized guidance.

d. **Stress Management:**

- Mindfulness and Relaxation Techniques: Practices such as meditation, yoga, and deep-breathing exercises can help reduce stress, which is known to impact blood pressure. Finding time for hobbies, socializing, and relaxation is also crucial.
- Support Systems: Building strong social networks and seeking support from family and friends can help individuals manage stress more effectively.

2. **Medical Interventions**

a. Regular Monitoring:
- Home Blood Pressure Monitoring: Regularly monitoring blood pressure at home can help individuals stay informed about their levels and the effectiveness of lifestyle changes. Keeping a log of readings can assist healthcare providers in tailoring treatment plans.

b. Medication Adherence:
- For some individuals, lifestyle changes alone may not suffice in managing hypertension, and medication may be necessary. It's essential to follow healthcare providers' recommendations regarding medications, including understanding dosages, potential side effects, and interactions.

Types of Medications:

- Common antihypertensive medications include diuretics, ACE inhibitors, calcium channel blockers, and beta-blockers. Each class works differently, and a healthcare provider will determine the best choice based on individual needs.

c. Regular Check-Ups:
- Maintaining regular appointments with healthcare providers allows for ongoing assessment and adjustment of treatment plans as needed. These check-ups can help address any concerns and reinforce the importance of adherence to lifestyle changes and medications.

3. **Community and Social Support**

a. Community Health Programs:
   - Participating in community health programs that focus on education, prevention, and support for hypertension can be beneficial. These programs may include workshops, support groups, and fitness classes tailored to individuals with hypertension.

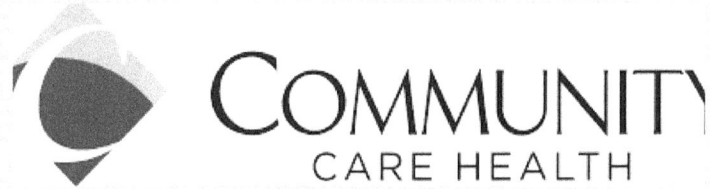

b. Educational Resources:
- Accessing educational materials from trusted organizations can empower individuals to make informed decisions about their health. Community centers, libraries, and online platforms can provide valuable resources about hypertension management.

c. Peer Support:
- Connecting with others who are managing hypertension can foster a sense of community and encourage. Support groups can facilitate sharing experiences, challenges, and strategies for success.

4. **Workplace Initiatives**

a. Employer-Led Health Programs:
- Workplaces can implement health programs that promote wellness, such as health screenings, fitness challenges, and educational workshops on managing hypertension. Employers may also offer incentives for employees who engage in healthy behaviors.

b. Flexible Work Environments:
- Providing flexible work arrangements can reduce stress and allow individuals to prioritize their health. Encouraging regular breaks and promoting a healthy work-life balance can contribute to overall well-being.

5. **Policy and Advocacy**

a. Public Health Initiatives:
- Advocating for policies that promote healthy environments—such as improved access to healthy foods, safe spaces for physical activity, and affordable healthcare—can have a lasting impact on hypertension prevention and management.

b. Awareness Campaigns:
- Supporting public awareness campaigns can enhance community knowledge about hypertension and encourage individuals to engage in preventive measures. Campaigns can focus on risk factors, the importance of monitoring, and lifestyle changes.

Conclusion

Preventing and managing hypertension requires a multifaceted approach that incorporates lifestyle modifications, medical interventions, community support, and advocacy. By empowering individuals with the tools and knowledge to take charge of their health, we can reduce the prevalence of hypertension and its associated complications. Collective efforts from individuals, healthcare providers, communities, and policymakers are essential in creating a healthier society.

Chapter IX
Future Directions in Hypertension Management

As our understanding of hypertension evolves, so too do the strategies for its management. Advances in research, technology, and healthcare practices are paving the way for more effective prevention and treatment approaches. This section explores the future directions in hypertension management, focusing on innovation, personalized care, and global initiatives.

1. **Personalized Medicine**

a. Genomic Insights:
  - Advances in genomics are transforming how we understand and treat hypertension. Genetic research is uncovering specific genetic markers associated with hypertension, enabling healthcare providers to tailor treatments based on an individual's genetic profile. This personalized approach aims to improve treatment efficacy and reduce side effects.

b. **Biomarkers and Risk Assessment:**

- The identification of biomarkers—biological indicators of disease—can enhance risk assessment for hypertension. These biomarkers may help predict an individual's response to specific medications or their likelihood of developing hypertension, leading to more targeted interventions.

c. Customized Treatment Plans:
- Personalized medicine encourages healthcare providers to develop individualized treatment plans that consider a patient's lifestyle, genetic factors, and preferences. This approach enhances patient engagement and adherence, ultimately leading to better health outcomes.

2. **Technological Innovations**

a. Telehealth Services:
  - Telehealth is revolutionizing hypertension management by providing remote access to healthcare providers. Patients can monitor their blood pressure at home and communicate with their doctors through virtual consultations. This model increases accessibility, particularly for individuals in remote or underserved areas.

b. Wearable Technology:
  - Wearable devices, such as smartwatches and fitness trackers, are increasingly being utilized to monitor vital signs, including blood pressure. These devices can provide real-time data, enabling patients to track their health metrics and share them with healthcare providers.

c. **Mobile Health Applications:**

- Mobile health (mHealth) apps are being developed to assist individuals in managing hypertension. These apps can offer features such as medication reminders, blood pressure tracking, and educational resources, empowering users to take an active role in their health.

3. Community-Based Approaches

a. **Health Promotion Initiatives:**

- Community-based health promotion initiatives are critical for raising awareness about hypertension and encouraging preventive measures. These programs can leverage local resources to provide education, screenings, and support in familiar settings.

b. **Collaborative Care Models:**

- Future hypertension management may increasingly adopt collaborative care models, involving multidisciplinary teams of healthcare providers—such as doctors, nurses, dietitians, and mental health professionals—to address the various factors contributing to hypertension. This holistic approach ensures comprehensive care tailored to individual needs.

c. Peer Support Networks:
- Establishing peer support networks within communities can foster shared experiences and encouragement among individuals managing hypertension. These networks can provide emotional support and practical tips for lifestyle changes and treatment adherence.

4. **Policy and Advocacy Efforts**

a. Public Health Campaigns:
- Advocacy for public health campaigns focused on hypertension prevention and management will be vital. These campaigns can raise awareness about risk factors, promote healthy lifestyles, and encourage regular blood pressure monitoring.

b. Addressing Health Disparities:
- Future initiatives must prioritize addressing health disparities in hypertension prevalence and treatment access. Policymakers and health organizations should work to ensure equitable access to healthcare resources and education for all populations, particularly marginalized communities.

c. **Global Collaboration:**

- Hypertension is a global health issue that requires international collaboration. Sharing research, resources, and successful intervention strategies across borders can enhance global efforts to combat hypertension and improve health outcomes.
-

5. **Ongoing Research and Innovation**
a. Exploring New Treatments:
- Research continues to explore new pharmacological treatments and innovative therapies for hypertension management. Investigating the potential of novel compounds, combination therapies, and alternative approaches can expand treatment options for patients.

b. **Behavioral Science Insights:**

- Understanding the behavioral and psychological factors that influence hypertension management is crucial. Future research may focus on developing interventions that leverage behavioral science to enhance adherence to lifestyle changes and medication regimens.

c. **Continuous Monitoring and Feedback:**

- Advancements in technology will enable continuous monitoring of blood pressure and other health indicators, allowing for real-time feedback and timely interventions. This proactive approach can help prevent complications and improve overall management.

Conclusion

The future of hypertension management is bright, driven by advances in personalized medicine, technology, community engagement, and policy initiatives. By embracing these innovations and fostering collaboration among healthcare providers, patients, and communities, we can create a comprehensive and effective approach to managing hypertension. Together, we can work toward reducing the burden of this chronic condition and improving health outcomes for individuals worldwide.

Chapter X

Advocacy and Policy Change

Advocacy and policy change play pivotal roles in addressing the challenges posed by hypertension. By influencing health policies and promoting public awareness, advocates can drive initiatives that improve prevention, treatment, and overall health outcomes. This section explores the significance of advocacy, strategies for effective change, and the role of various stakeholders in combating hypertension.

1. **The Importance of Advocacy**

a. Raising Awareness:
- Advocacy efforts are essential for raising public and governmental awareness about the prevalence and impact of hypertension. By highlighting the condition's seriousness, advocates can foster a sense of urgency and promote action at local, national, and global levels.

b. Educating Stakeholders:
- Advocates play a crucial role in educating healthcare providers, policymakers, and the general public about hypertension, its risk factors, and the importance of prevention and management strategies. This education can lead to informed decision-making and policy formulation.

c. **Empowering Patients:**

- Advocacy initiatives empower individuals with hypertension by providing resources, information, and support. By encouraging patients to share their experiences and advocate for their needs, these initiatives help amplify their voices in the healthcare system.

2. Strategies for Effective Advocacy

a. Building Coalitions:
- Forming coalitions with healthcare organizations, community groups, and advocacy organizations can amplify efforts. Collaborating on initiatives, campaigns, and educational programs allows for a broader reach and a unified message.

b. **Engaging in Grassroots Campaigns:**

- Grassroots campaigns mobilize community members to advocate for hypertension awareness and policy changes. These efforts can include organizing events, conducting health fairs, and leveraging social media to raise awareness and encourage community involvement.

c. Utilizing Data and Research:
- Evidence-based advocacy is crucial for effecting change. Utilizing data on hypertension prevalence, healthcare costs, and health outcomes can strengthen advocacy messages and support policy recommendations. Research findings can help demonstrate the need for effective interventions and resources.

3. **Policy Change Initiatives**

a. Promoting Access to Care:
- Advocates can push for policies that improve access to hypertension screening, treatment, and management resources. This may involve advocating for insurance coverage for preventive services, medications, and educational programs.

b. Supporting Healthy Environments:
- Policy changes that promote healthy environments—such as improving access to nutritious foods, safe spaces for physical activity, and smoke-free areas—are essential for hypertension prevention. Advocates can work with local governments to implement policies that foster healthy community conditions.

c. Funding for Research and Programs:
- Securing funding for research initiatives and community health programs focused on hypertension is vital. Advocates can lobby for public funding and grants to support evidence-based programs that address the burden of hypertension.

4. **The Role of Healthcare Professionals**

a. Engaging Healthcare Providers:
- Healthcare professionals can serve as powerful advocates for their patients and communities. By educating colleagues about hypertension management and advocating for systemic changes within healthcare systems, providers can drive improvements in care delivery.

b. Incorporating Advocacy into Practice:
- Integrating advocacy into clinical practice involves discussing the importance of hypertension management with patients and encouraging them to participate in advocacy efforts. Healthcare providers can help patients understand their role in driving change and seeking support.

5. **Global Perspective on Advocacy**

a. International Collaboration:
- Hypertension is a global health issue, and advocacy efforts should transcend borders. Collaborating with international organizations, such as the World Health Organization (WHO) and the International Society of Hypertension (ISH), can facilitate knowledge sharing and promote global health initiatives.

b. Addressing Health Disparities:
- Advocacy must focus on addressing health disparities in hypertension prevalence and management. Ensuring that marginalized and underserved populations receive adequate support and resources is essential for promoting equity in healthcare.

6. **Measuring Advocacy Impact**

a. Evaluating Effectiveness:
- Assessing the impact of advocacy initiatives is crucial for understanding their effectiveness. This can involve tracking changes in public awareness, healthcare access, and health outcomes related to hypertension.

b. Adjusting Strategies:
- Continuous evaluation allows advocates to adjust strategies based on feedback and results. By identifying successful approaches and areas for improvement, advocates can refine their efforts for greater impact.

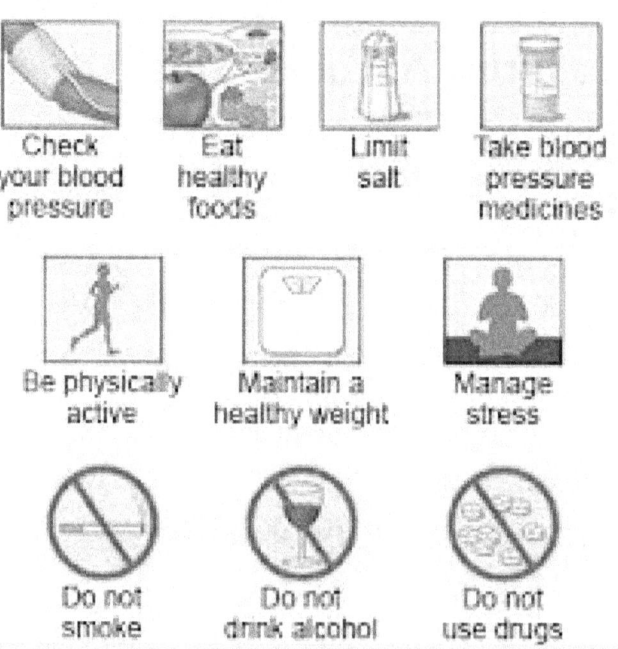

Conclusion

Advocacy and policy change are essential components in the fight against hypertension. By raising awareness, promoting access to care, and influencing policy decisions, advocates can drive meaningful change in hypertension management. Collaborative efforts among individuals, healthcare providers, and organizations are key to creating a healthier future for all, where hypertension is effectively prevented and managed. Through sustained advocacy, we can work towards a society that prioritizes heart health and empowers individuals to take charge of their well-being.

Conclusion
The Path Forward

As we conclude this exploration of hypertension and its multifaceted impact on society, it is clear that addressing this pervasive condition requires a collective effort from individuals, healthcare providers, communities, and policymakers. Hypertension is not merely a personal health issue; it is a public health challenge that demands a comprehensive and proactive approach.

1. **Summary of Key Points**

Throughout this ebook, we have delved into various aspects of hypertension, including its definitions, classifications, risk factors, cultural perspectives, awareness and education, prevention and management strategies, future directions, advocacy, and policy change. Each chapter has highlighted the complexity of hypertension and underscored the importance of understanding the interplay between lifestyle, genetics, environment, and healthcare access.

2. The Importance of Awareness and Education

Increasing awareness and education about hypertension remains paramount. By empowering individuals with knowledge about their health, we can foster a culture of prevention. Comprehensive education initiatives, tailored to diverse populations, can enhance understanding of risk factors, symptoms, and management strategies, ultimately leading to earlier detection and better health outcomes.

3. **Embracing Prevention and Lifestyle Changes**

Preventive measures are essential in combating hypertension. Encouraging healthy lifestyle changes—such as adopting a balanced diet, engaging in regular physical activity, managing stress, and maintaining a healthy weight—can significantly reduce the incidence of hypertension. Communities, healthcare providers, and individuals must work together to create supportive environments that promote these healthy behaviors.

4. Innovations in Management and Treatment

The future of hypertension management is promising, with advancements in personalized medicine, technology, and community engagement. Telehealth services, wearable devices, and mobile health applications are transforming how individuals monitor and manage their blood pressure. As we embrace these innovations, it is vital to ensure that all individuals have access to these resources, regardless of their socioeconomic status or geographic location.

5. The Role of Advocacy and Policy Change

Advocacy and policy change are crucial for creating systemic improvements in hypertension management. By advocating for policies that enhance access to healthcare, promote healthy environments, and support research initiatives, we can address the root causes of hypertension and promote equity in healthcare access. Collaboration among healthcare providers, community organizations, and policymakers will be essential in driving these efforts.

6. A Call to Action

Addressing hypertension is a shared responsibility that requires commitment and action from all sectors of society. Individuals must take charge of their health, healthcare providers must continue to educate and support their patients, and communities must advocate for resources and policies that promote wellness. Together, we can build a healthier future where hypertension is effectively managed, and individuals are empowered to lead fulfilling lives.

7. **Looking Ahead**

As we move forward, ongoing research and innovation will be vital in uncovering new insights into hypertension and developing more effective prevention and treatment strategies. By fostering a culture of collaboration, we can harness the power of diverse perspectives and expertise to create meaningful change. In conclusion, while the challenges posed by hypertension are significant, they are not insurmountable. By working together and prioritizing heart health, we can pave the way for a healthier society, reduce the burden of hypertension, and improve the quality of life for millions around the world. Let us commit to this path forward with determination and hope.

Resources and Further Reading

1. Books:
   - "Hypertension: A Companion to Braunwald's Heart Disease" by George L. Bakris and Matthew Sorrentino
     - A comprehensive guide covering the pathophysiology, diagnosis, and treatment of hypertension.
   - "The DASH Diet Action Plan" by Marla Heller
     - A practical guide to adopting the DASH diet for lowering blood pressure.
   - "Understanding High Blood Pressure" by J. D. C. Matz
     - An accessible resource that explains hypertension in layman's terms.

Websites:

- American Heart Association: www.heart.org
    - Offers resources on heart health, including hypertension management and prevention tips.
- Centers for Disease Control and Prevention (CDC): www.cdc.gov
    - Provides information on public health initiatives related to hypertension and heart disease.
- National Heart, Lung, and Blood Institute (NHLBI): www.nhlbi.nih.gov
    - A comprehensive source for research, guidelines, and education materials on heart health.

Research Journals:

- Hypertension (Journal of the American Heart Association)
    - Features the latest research on hypertension, including studies on treatment and management.
- Journal of Clinical Hypertension
    - Publishes research, reviews, and clinical guidelines related to hypertension and its management.

- **Videos and Documentaries:**

- TED Talks on health and wellness, featuring experts discussing heart health and hypertension.
- YouTube Channels like the American Heart Association offer informative videos about managing hypertension.
- Support and Advocacy Organizations:
- The American Society of Hypertension (ASH): www.ash-us.org
    - Provides resources for healthcare professionals and patients, including guidelines and research updates.
- Blood Pressure UK: www.bloodpressureuk.org
    - Offers support, information, and resources specifically for individuals dealing with hypertension.

References

- American Heart Association. (2023). Hypertension: A Public Health Perspective. Retrieved from www.heart.org
- Mills, K. T., Bundy, J. D., Kelly, T. N., et al. (2016). Global disparities of hypertension prevalence and control: a systematic analysis of worldwide data. Lancet, 387(10024), 10012-10024. doi:10.1016/S0140-6736(15)01253-2
- Kearney, P. M., Whelton, M., Reynolds, K., et al. (2005). Global burden of hypertension: analysis of worldwide data. Lancet, 365(9455), 217-223. doi:10.1016/S0140-6736(05)17741-1
- Sacks, F. M., Svetkey, L. P., Vollmer, W. M., et al. (2001). Effects on blood pressure of reduced dietary sodium and the Dietary Approaches to Stop Hypertension (DASH) diet. New England Journal of Medicine, 344(1), 3-10. doi:10.1056/NEJM200101043440101
- Whelton, P. K., Carey, R. M., Aronow, W. S., et al. (2018). 2017 Guideline for the Prevention, Detection, Evaluation, and Management of High Blood Pressure in Adults. Hypertension, 71(6), e13-e115. doi:10.1161/HYP.0000000000000065
- Centers for Disease Control and Prevention (CDC). (2021). High Blood Pressure Facts. Retrieved from www.cdc.gov

- World Health Organization (WHO). (2022). Hypertension. Retrieved from www.who.int
- Nishiyama, A., & Yoshida, K. (2017). Renal sympathetic nerve activity and hypertension: mechanisms and therapeutic implications. Nature Reviews Nephrology, 13(4), 207-220. doi:10.1038/nrneph.2017.3
- Boden-Albala, B., Litvak, E., & Ramaswamy, R. (2008). Hypertension, hyperlipidemia, and diabetes: The role of health literacy. Journal of Clinical Hypertension, 10(8), 572-578. doi:10.1111/j.1751-7176.2008.08543.x
- Meyer, S., & Mattes, R. D. (2020). The impact of dietary patterns on blood pressure: A systematic review. American Journal of Hypertension, 33(8), 785-793. doi:10.1093/ajh/hpaa038
- National Heart, Lung, and Blood Institute (NHLBI). (2023). What Is High Blood Pressure? Retrieved from www.nhlbi.nih.gov
- Kahn, S. E., Cooper, M. E., & Del Prato, S. (2014). Pathophysiology and treatment of type 2 diabetes: perspectives on the past, present, and future. Lancet, 383(9924), 1069-1080. doi:10.1016/S0140-6736(13)62154-6

www.ingramcontent.com/pod-product-compliance
Lightning Source LLC
Chambersburg PA
CBHW070151230526
45471CB00002B/615